# HEALTHY GUIDE TO GLOWING AS YOU AGE

## Proven strategies to staying young and active as you get older

**NGOZIA WELLS**

# DISCLAIMER

Disclaimer: The information provided in this "healthy guide to glowing as you age" is intended for general educational and informational purposes only. It is not a substitute for professional medical advice, diagnosis, or treatment. Always consult with a qualified healthcare provider before making any changes to your diet, exercise routine, or healthcare regimen.

# DEDICATION

I dedicate to my lovely husband Pastor Ethel Osthia who has been of immense support all through the process of writing this book

To my children for being there.

# INTRODUCTION

Aging is a natural process that everyone goes through, However, it's possible to age gracefully and maintain a youthful glow by taking care of our health and well-being. A healthy guide to glowing as you age involves adopting a healthy lifestyle that includes proper nutrition, regular exercise, stress management, and self-care. These practices can help you maintain healthy skin, strong muscles and bones, a sharp mind and a positive outlook on life as you age. Additionally, the guide may also include tips on skincare, sleep habits, and other healthy habits that can contribute to your overall well-being. By following these healthy practices, you can embrace aging with grace and confidence, and enjoy a healthy and vibrant life for years to come.

# CHAPTER ONE

## IMPORTANCE OF NUTRITION FOR HEALTHY AGEING

As we age, our bodies go through a number of changes that can have an impact on our overall health and well-being. One of the most important factors that can influence healthy ageing is nutrition. Good nutrition is essential for maintaining good health, and it becomes even more important as we get older.

Here are some key reasons why nutrition is important for healthy ageing:

Maintaining a Healthy Weight: As we age, our metabolism slows down, and we may find it more difficult to maintain a healthy weight. A diet that is high in nutrient-dense foods, such as fruits, vegetables, whole grains, lean proteins, and healthy fats, can help to keep us feeling full and satisfied, while also providing the necessary vitamins and minerals that our bodies need to function properly.

Reducing the Risk of Chronic Diseases: A healthy diet can help to reduce the risk of chronic diseases such as heart disease, stroke, diabetes, and certain types of cancer. By choosing foods that are rich in antioxidants, fiber, and other nutrients, we can help to protect our bodies against damage caused by free radicals, reduce inflammation, and promote overall health and well-being.

Boosting Immunity: A healthy diet can also help to boost the immune system, which can help to protect against illness and disease. By choosing foods that are rich in vitamins and minerals, such as vitamin C, zinc, and selenium, we can help to support a healthy immune system.

Improving Cognitive Function: Good nutrition is also important for maintaining cognitive function and reducing the risk of cognitive decline. A diet that is rich in omega-3 fatty acids, antioxidants, and other nutrients can help to protect against age-related cognitive decline and improve brain function.

In summary, nutrition plays a vital role in healthy ageing. By choosing a diet that is rich in nutrient-dense foods and essential vitamins and minerals, we can help to maintain good health, reduce the risk of chronic diseases, and improve overall well-being as we age.

# CHAPTER TWO

## REGULAR EXERCISE FOR HEALTHY GLOW

Regular exercise is not just good for your physical health, but it can also have a significant impact on your skin's appearance. Here are some ways that regular exercise can give you a youthful glow

Increased Blood Flow: Exercise increases blood flow throughout your body, including your skin. This increased circulation helps to deliver oxygen and nutrients to your skin cells, which can make your skin look healthier and more radiant.

Reduced Stress: Exercise is a great way to reduce stress, and stress can have a negative impact on your skin's appearance. When you're stressed, your body produces cortisol, a hormone that can lead to acne, wrinkles, and other skin problems. Regular exercise can help to reduce cortisol levels and promote healthy skin.

Improved Skin Elasticity: Exercise can also help to improve your skin's elasticity. As you age, your skin loses elasticity, which can lead to wrinkles and sagging. By exercising regularly, you can help to improve your skin's elasticity and reduce the signs of aging.

Increased Collagen Production: Collagen is a protein that gives your skin its elasticity and firmness. Your body generates less collagen as you get older, which can cause wrinkles and drooping skin. Exercise can help to stimulate collagen production, which can make your skin look more youthful and vibrant.

Reduced Inflammation: Chronic inflammation can have a negative impact on your skin's appearance. Regular exercise can help to reduce inflammation throughout your body, which can help to improve the appearance of your skin.

Improved Blood Circulation: Exercise increases blood flow, which provides oxygen and nutrients to the skin cells, helping them to function more effectively. It also removes waste products from the skin cells, making the skin look clearer and healthier.

Detoxification: Exercise helps to flush out toxins from the body through sweating, which can help to keep the skin clear and healthy-looking. For those with skin prone to acne, this may be very helpful.

Improved Sleep: Regular exercise has been shown to improve sleep quality, which can have a positive impact on the skin. During sleep, the body produces growth hormones that help to repair and regenerate skin cells, resulting in a brighter and more youthful-looking complexion.

To achieve a youthful glow through exercise, it is recommended to engage in moderate-intensity exercise for at least 30 minutes, five times a week. This might entail engaging in exercise like jogging, cycling, swimming, or dancing. To maintain good skin, it's also crucial to keep hydrated by drinking enough of water before, during, and after exercise. Moreover, shielding yourself from the sun's rays with clothing and sunscreen when engaging in outdoor activities will delay skin aging.

In conclusion, regular exercise can have a significant impact on your skin's appearance, helping you to achieve a more youthful and radiant glow. So, if you want to look and feel your best, make sure to incorporate regular exercise into your daily routine

# CHAPTER THREE

## SLEEP AND ITS ROLE IN ANTI-AGING

Sleep plays a crucial role in anti-aging by allowing the body to repair, regenerate, and rejuvenate itself. When we sleep, the body goes through a series of processes that help repair and restore our cells, tissues, and organs. Lack of sleep or poor quality sleep can accelerate the aging process and lead to a variety of health problems, including premature aging.

One of the main ways that sleep contributes to anti-aging is by promoting the production of human growth hormone (HGH). HGH is a hormone that is responsible for cell growth, metabolism, and regeneration. It is released by the pituitary gland during sleep, particularly during deep, slow-wave sleep. HGH helps to repair and regenerate cells throughout the body, including the skin, muscles, bones, and organs.

In addition to promoting the production of HGH, sleep also helps to reduce inflammation in the body. Chronic inflammation is a major contributor to aging and age-related diseases such as arthritis, diabetes, and heart disease. Sleep helps to reduce inflammation by regulating the immune system and reducing the levels of stress hormones in the body.

Sleep also plays a role in maintaining the health and appearance of the skin. During sleep, the body produces collagen, a protein that helps to keep the skin firm, elastic, and wrinkle-free. Lack of sleep or poor quality sleep can lead to decreased collagen production, which can contribute to the development of wrinkles, fine lines, and other signs of aging.

Sleep reduces inflammation: Chronic inflammation is a major contributor to aging and age-related diseases. Lack of sleep or poor quality sleep can lead to increased inflammation in the body. Inflammation is linked to a variety of health problems, including arthritis, diabetes, heart disease, and cancer. Sleep helps to regulate the immune system and reduce the levels of stress hormones in the body, which helps to reduce inflammation.

Sleep maintains skin health: Collagen is a protein that helps to keep the skin firm, elastic, and wrinkle-free. During sleep, the body produces collagen, which helps to repair and regenerate the skin. Lack of sleep or poor quality sleep can lead to decreased collagen production, which can contribute to the development of wrinkles, fine lines, and other signs of aging. In addition, sleep helps to regulate the levels of cortisol, a hormone that can contribute to skin aging.

Sleep improves cognitive function and memory: Cognitive function and memory can decline with age. During sleep, the brain consolidates and processes memories, which helps to improve learning and retention. Sleep also plays a role in regulating mood and emotions, which can be affected by aging-related changes in brain function. Getting enough quality sleep is essential for maintaining optimal cognitive function and preventing cognitive decline.

Sleep improves overall health: Lack of sleep or poor quality sleep is linked to a variety of health problems, including obesity, diabetes, heart disease, and depression. Getting enough quality sleep is essential for maintaining overall health and preventing premature aging.

Sleep helps to improve cognitive function and memory, which can decline with age. During sleep, the brain consolidates and processes memories, which helps to improve learning and retention. Sleep also plays a role in regulating mood and emotions, which can be affected by aging-related changes in brain function.

In conclusion, sleep plays a critical role in anti-aging by promoting the production of HGH, reducing inflammation, maintaining skin health, improving cognitive function and memory, and improving overall health. Getting enough quality sleep is essential for maintaining optimal health and preventing premature aging. It is recommended that adults get 7-9 hours of sleep per night to maintain optimal health and prevent premature aging.

# CHAPTER FOUR.

## MANAGING STRESS FOR A HEALTHY MIND AND BODY.

Life is full of stress, which is expected. Depression can stem from several things, including employment, relationships, problems with money, or one's health. Chronic stress can have detrimental consequences on our mind and body, although some stress is acceptable and even helpful in short quantities. The following are some techniques for reducing stress and enhancing general health and well-being:

Exercise: One of the best ways to alleviate stress is through regular exercise. Workout releases natural mood enhancers called endorphins. It also aids in easing muscle tension, which can lessen the physical effects of stress.

Try relaxation techniques: Deep breathing, meditation, and progressive muscle relaxation are just a few of the methods that can help you unwind and reduce stress.

Get enough rest: Sleep deprivation can lead to stress and make it more difficult to handle challenging circumstances. Strive for 7-9 hours of sleep each night to support both physical and mental well-being.

Practice self-care: Making time for leisure activities can assist to lower stress and enhance general well-being. This could involve pastimes, quality time with loved ones, or even just a soothing bath.

Managing your time: Having too much to accomplish and not enough time to get it done can lead to feelings of overload and tension. Making a timetable and setting priorities might help you better manage your time and feel less stressed.

Interact with others: Social support is a potent stress-reduction technique. Joining a support group or spending time with friends and family can offer emotional support and a sense of community.

Consume well-balanced meals that are high in fruits, vegetables, whole grains, and lean protein to help you stay healthy generally and relieve stress.

Avoid using unhealthy coping strategies: While it may seem alluring to use a drink, drugs, or other unhealthy coping strategies to deal with stress, doing so can end up making matters worse in the long run. Instead, concentrate on wholesome coping mechanisms that encourage unwinding and well-being.

It's crucial to identify what works best for you because everyone feels stress in various ways. These techniques can be incorporated into your everyday routine to help you manage stress and encourage both mental and physical wellness.

Set self-reflection as a top priority. By taking the time to think about your feelings and thoughts, you can learn where your stress comes from and how to handle it.

Take pauses: You may stay focused and recharge by taking little breaks throughout the day. This could be going for a brief stroll, enjoying some music, or practicing some rapid meditation techniques.

Get organized: Clutter and disarray can heighten stress and overwhelm feelings. Decluttering and organizing your space might make you feel calmer and more concentrated.

Cultivate gratitude: Spending some time each day thinking about what you have to be thankful for might help you become more optimistic and relieve tension and anxiety.

Get in touch with your basic values: Being in touch with your core values might help you keep perspective and concentrate on what is essential. Feelings of stress and overwhelm may be lessened as a result.

Engage in constructive communication: Developing strong communication skills will assist you in controlling relationship stress and preventing conflict from escalating.

Establishing sound limits can aid in stress management and the avoidance of burnout. This can entail limiting your work hours or declining commitments that conflict with your priorities.

Exercise self-compassion: Being understanding and kind to yourself can aid in resilience building and stress management. Take into account the fact that everyone makes errors and has terrible days.

Laugh and have fun: Making time for enjoyment-inducing activities can help lower stress levels and enhance general well-being.

# CHAPTER FIVE

## THE ADVANTAGES OF SKIN CARE FOR AGING SKIN.

Many advantages of anti-aging skin care include:

Reduction in the visibility of fine lines and wrinkles: Skin care products and treatments made especially for aging skin can help minimize the visibility of lines and wrinkles, giving the skin a smoother, more youthful appearance.

Better skin texture: Using skin care products regularly may help make older skin seem smoother, softer, and more supple.

Improved hydration: As we become older, our skin dries up and becomes more prone to wrinkles. Keeping the skin moisturized and minimizing the appearance of dryness may be achieved by using moisturizers and other hydrating treatments.

Prevention from sun damage: Using products with SPF can help shield the skin from damaging UV rays, which can cause premature aging and wrinkles.

skin tone is more even: Aged skin sometimes appears dull and uneven in tone. Frequent application of skin care products containing retinol and vitamin C can assist to enhance the overall tone and radiance of the skin.

increased collagen synthesis: Collagen, a protein that keeps skin elastic and tight, is produced at a higher rate. We produce less natural collagen as we get older, which causes sagging and wrinkles.

Some components in skin care products have the potential to increase the formation of collagen, which can help improve the look of aged skin.

In general, maintaining aged skin with a regular skin care regimen can benefit the skin's look, texture, and general health, as well as slow the aging process.

# CHAPTER SIX

## SUN PROTECTION FOR PREVENTING WRINKLES

Although wrinkles are a normal aspect of getting older, too much sun exposure can hasten the aging process and cause premature wrinkles. One of the best strategies to stop wrinkles and keep healthy, youthful-looking skin is sun protection.

Here are some suggestions for sun protection and wrinkle prevention for your skin:

Use sunscreen: Applying sunscreen is the most crucial step you can do to protect your skin from the sun. Choose a broad-spectrum sunscreen that has an SPF of at least 30, then liberally apply it to your hands, neck, face, and any other exposed skin. Every two hours after swimming or perspiring, reapply.

Seek Shade: During the height of the sun's rays, seek shade whenever you can (10 a.m. to 4 p.m.). As a result, you'll be exposed to fewer UV rays overall and have a lower chance of getting wrinkles and other sun damage.

Wear Sun-Protective Clothes: Wear long-sleeved shirts, long pants, and hats with broad brims to protect yourself from the sun. This will lessen your chance of wrinkle development and protect your skin from the sun.

Avoid Tanning: While it can be alluring to tan, especially during the summer, doing so can raise your risk of wrinkles and other age indicators. Instead, if you want to seem sun-kissed, choose a self-tanner or bronzer.

Employ skincare products that contain antioxidants: Antioxidants can help shield your skin from free radical damage, which can exacerbate wrinkles and other aging symptoms. Try to choose skincare products that have antioxidants like green tea, vitamin C, and vitamin E.

Keep Hydrated: Consuming lots of water will keep your skin healthy and moisturized, which can lower your risk of wrinkles. To assist retain moisture, try to consume at least 8 glasses of water each day and think about applying a moisturizer.

In conclusion, one of the most crucial things you can do to avoid wrinkles and maintain healthy, youthful-looking skin is to protect your skin from the sun. You can lessen your risk of getting wrinkles and other aging symptoms by heeding these recommendations and prioritizing sun protection.

# CHAPTER SEVEN

## HYDRATION FOR GLOWING SKIN

Hydration for Glowing Skin is essential for maintaining healthy, glowing skin. The cells that make up our skin need water to function properly. When our skin is dehydrated, it can look dull, dry, and lackluster. In this article, we'll explore the important roles hydration plays in achieving glowing skin and how to ensure our skin stays hydrated.

Hydration is essential for maintaining healthy, glowing skin. Our skin is made up of cells that require water to function properly. When our skin is dehydrated, it can look dull, dry, and lackluster. In this article, we'll explore the important roles hydration plays in achieving glowing skin and how to ensure our skin stays hydrated.

Moisturizing:

Hydration is critical to maintaining the skin's moisture barrier, which helps lock in moisture and prevent water loss. When our skin is dehydrated, it can cause the skin to overproduce oil, leading to breakouts and an uneven skin texture. Moisturizing your skin with a hydrating moisturizer can help replenish the skin's moisture barrier and prevent water loss, resulting in a plump, radiant complexion.

Elasticity:

Skin elasticity refers to the skin's ability to bounce back after being stretched or pulled. When our skin is hydrated, it becomes more elastic, which can help reduce the appearance of fine lines and wrinkles. Dehydrated skin, on the other hand, can make wrinkles and fine lines more visible, leading to a tired, aged appearance.

Blood circulation:

Hydration also plays a role in maintaining healthy blood circulation in the skin. When our skin is well-hydrated, blood can flow more easily, delivering essential nutrients and oxygen to the skin cells. This can help improve skin tone and texture, giving the skin a healthy, youthful glow.

Detoxification:

Our skin acts as a barrier to protect us from harmful toxins and pollutants. When our skin is hydrated, it can more effectively eliminate toxins through sweat and other excretions, keeping our skin healthy and glowing.

In conclusion, hydration is vital for achieving and maintaining glowing, healthy skin. Drinking enough water and using hydrating skincare products can help keep our skin well-hydrated and protected from environmental stressors, leading to a more radiant complexion.

# CHAPTER EIGHT

## STIMULATION OF THE MIND FOR BRAIN HEALTH

The significance of mental exercise for brain health

Since it keeps the brain active and operating at its best, mental stimulation is crucial for brain health. Like any other muscle in the body, the brain needs regular training to be flexible and strong. Puzzles, reading, learning a new language, playing an instrument, and other cognitively demanding hobbies are just a few examples of activities that may stimulate the mind.

According to research, mental exercise can boost one's cognition, memory, and attention. Frequent mental exercise has been associated with a lower risk of Alzheimer's disease, dementia, and age-related cognitive decline.

Moreover, mental activity can enhance mood, lessen stress and anxiety, and boost general well-being. Also, it can give a sense of fulfillment and purpose, which can raise the overall quality of life.

It's crucial to remember that mental stimulation should be customized to a person's interests and skills. Taking part in hard yet non-stressful activities can support the best possible brain health. For total brain health, it's also critical to include social contact, a balanced diet, and physical activity in one's daily routine.

Enhanced Brain Plasticity: The brain's capacity to adapt and alter to new circumstances is known as brain plasticity. Enhancing brain plasticity through mental stimulation can help the brain better deal with damage or sickness and recover from it.

Improved Creativity: Taking part in cognitively challenging activities can foster the generation of fresh ideas and aid to increase creativity.

Decreased Risk of Depression: By encouraging the development of new brain cells and boosting the synthesis of neurotransmitters like serotonin and dopamine, mental stimulation can assist to lower the risk of depression.

Improved Productivity: Mentally stimulating activities can aid with attention and focus, which increases productivity and efficiency.

Delaying age-related cognitive decline can help people preserve their mental acuity and independence for a longer period. This is done by engaging in regular mental stimulation.

Increased Sleep Quality: By lowering stress and anxiety, encouraging relaxation, and boosting the synthesis of hormones that sleep aid, mental stimulation can assist to enhance sleep quality.

Improved Stress Management: By giving stress a constructive outlet, engaging in cognitively challenging activities can assist to enhance stress management.

# CHAPTER NINE

## AGE AND RELATIONSHIP

Strong connections are crucial at any stage of life, but as we become older, they can become more difficult to establish and sustain. Our living conditions, physical health, and social networks may alter as we become older. Yet it is possible to build and maintain meaningful connections throughout our lives with a little work and dedication. Here are some pointers for developing and preserving solid connections as you become older:

Place a high priority on communication because it is the cornerstone of any successful relationship. Prioritizing communication with the essential individuals in your life becomes even more crucial as you get older. Whether it be through phone conversations, video chats, or in-person visits, make an effort to remain in touch with loved ones frequently.

Discover shared interests: Hobbies and interests may be a terrific way to connect with others and sustain long-lasting connections. Becoming involved in organizations or organizations that share your interests may be a terrific opportunity to make new friends and meet new people.

Have an open mind: As you become older, it might be tempting to get into a habit and stay with what you know. But, being open to new experiences helps keep bonds intriguing and vibrant. Try new things with the people in your life, go on new adventures, and explore new locations.

Express your appreciation: Building and sustaining healthy connections may be facilitated by letting others know how much you value them and the things they do for you. Spend some time being thankful and appreciative of the people in your life.

Be patient: Building and maintaining relationships takes time and effort. As you manage the ups and downs of establishing and maintaining relationships, have patience with both yourself and other people.

Ask for aid when you need it; it's OK to do so. By seeking assistance, whether it comes from family, friends, or a professional, you may overcome obstacles and improve your connections.

You may develop and sustain successful connections as you age by emphasizing communication, discovering similar interests, being open to new experiences, exercising empathy, demonstrating gratitude, being patient, and asking for help when necessary.

# CHAPTER TEN

# HEALTH PREVENTION ACTIONS TO DECREASE CHRONIC DISEASE RISK

The risk of chronic illnesses must be reduced in large part by preventative health interventions. Globally, the major causes of mortality include chronic conditions such as diabetes, cancer, heart disease, stroke, and obesity. Lifestyle factors including poor diet, physical inactivity, smoking, and excessive alcohol intake are frequently to blame for these disorders. The following preventative health actions can help lower the chance of developing chronic diseases:

Healthy Eating: Preventing chronic illnesses requires a healthy diet. The risk of heart disease, stroke, diabetes, and some forms of cancer can be decreased by eating a diet high in fruits, vegetables, whole grains, lean meats, and healthy fats. Limiting the intake of processed meals, sweet beverages, and saturated and trans fats is crucial.

Avoiding Smoking: Chronic illnesses including lung cancer, heart disease, and stroke are mostly brought on by smoking. Smoking cessation can lower the chance of developing certain illnesses. Another key factor is avoiding exposure to secondhand smoke.

Limiting Alcohol Consumption: Chronic conditions including liver disease, cancer, and heart disease are all made more likely by excessive alcohol use. The risk of these illnesses can be decreased by limiting alcohol consumption to no more than one drink per day for women and two drinks per day for men.

Being Screened for Chronic Diseases: Treatment results can be improved by early identification of chronic diseases including cancer, diabetes, and high blood pressure. Receiving a screening for certain illnesses can aid in their early detection and enable early intervention and treatment.

Keeping a Healthy Weight: It's critical to keep a healthy weight to fend against chronic illnesses. Obesity and overweight can raise one's chance of developing heart disease, stroke, diabetes, and several cancers. Healthy eating habits and regular exercise can help people stay at a healthy weight, which lowers their chance of developing certain diseases.

In conclusion, maintaining total health and well-being requires preventing chronic illnesses via appropriate lifestyle decisions. You may lower your chance of developing chronic illnesses and have a better, happier life by implementing these preventative health steps into your everyday routine.